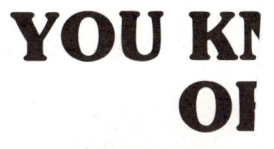

YOU KN
OI

MW01602224

DIET

WHEN....

*. . . it takes the whole neighborhood
to be your partner on a teeter-totter.*

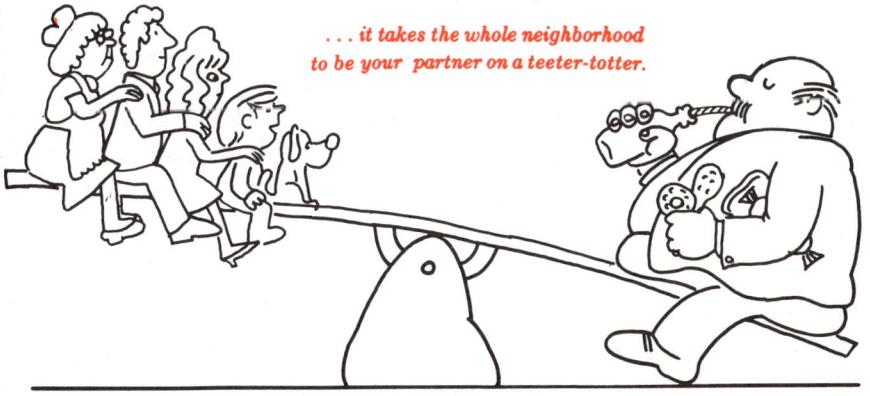

BY MARTIN A. RAGAWAY   ILLUSTRATIONS BY DON ROBB

a **Laughter Library** book

PRICE/STERN/SLOAN

Publishers, Inc., Los Angeles

1983

DEDICATION

*To those resourceful, devoted,
courageous, persevering, scrupulous
individuals who go to
any lengths to avoid
further width, this book
is optimistically dedicated.*

Copyright© 1983 by The Laughter Library
Published by Price/Stern/Sloan Publishers, Inc.
410 North La Cienega Boulevard, Los Angeles, California 90048

ISBN: 0-8431-0549-6

YOU KNOW YOU'RE OFF YOUR DIET WHEN · · · · · ·

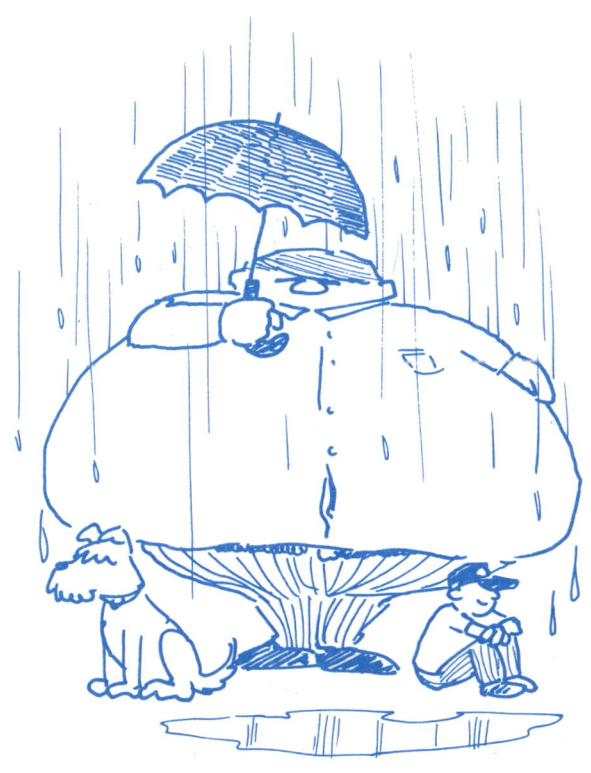

. . . it rains and nothing below your waist gets wet.

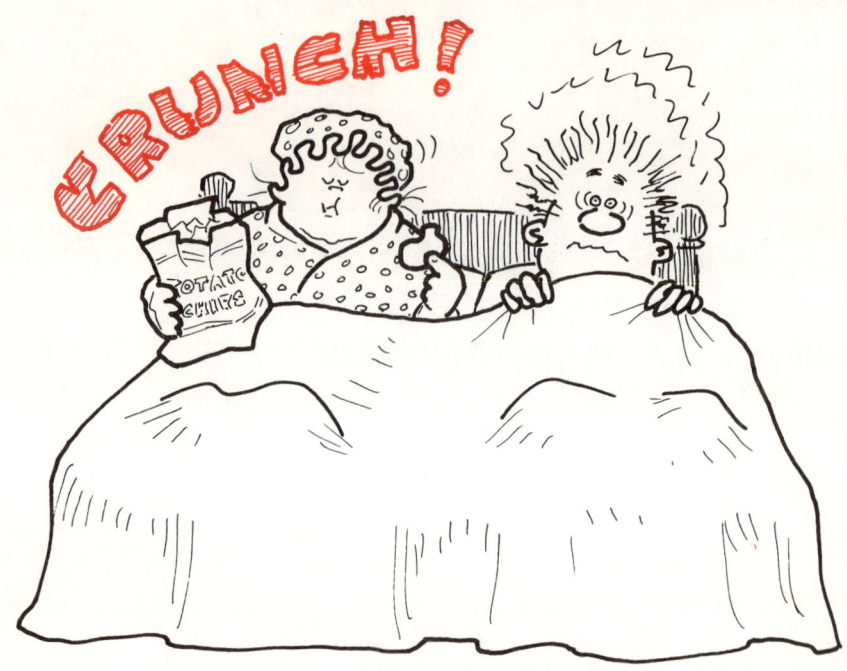

. . . you try to invent a noiseless potato chip, so in the middle of the night you can get away with cheating.

REFUSING SECONDS
IS NO HELP WHEN...

...you finally got it all together and you can't get it off.

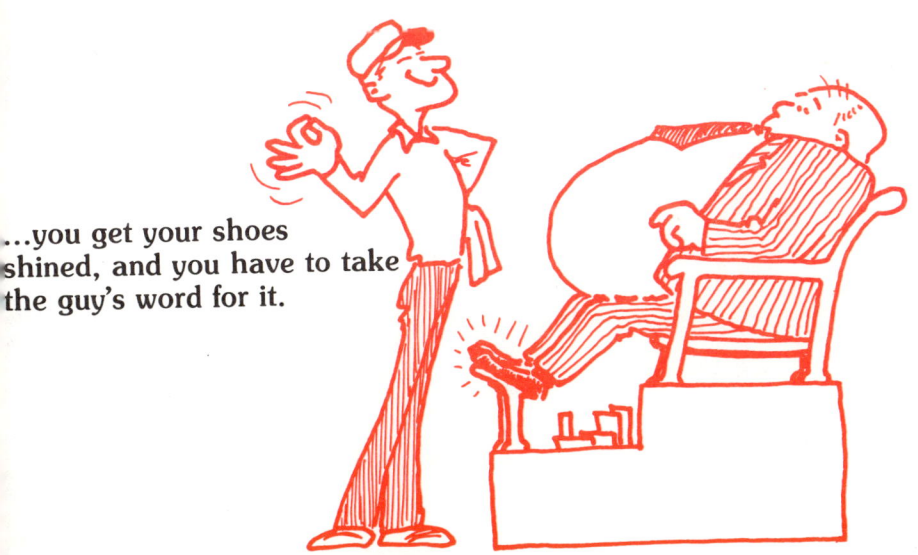

...you get your shoes shined, and you have to take the guy's word for it.

IT ISN'T YOUR BATH SCALE, IT'S <u>YOU</u> IF...

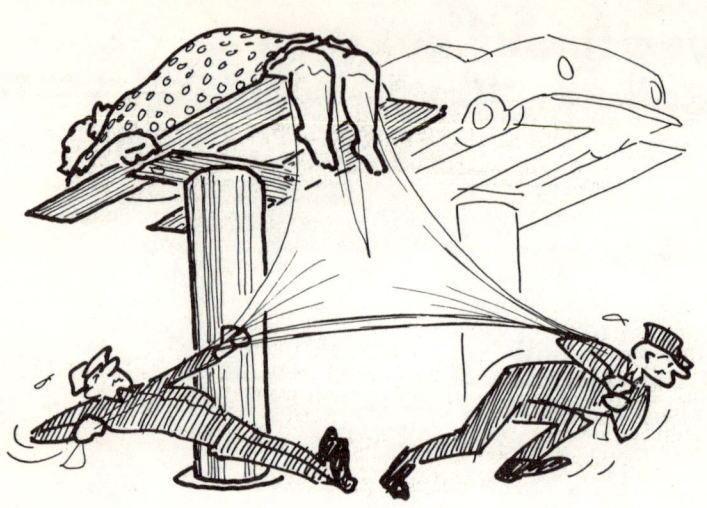

...to get your panty hose off, you have to go down to the service station and be put up on the grease rack.

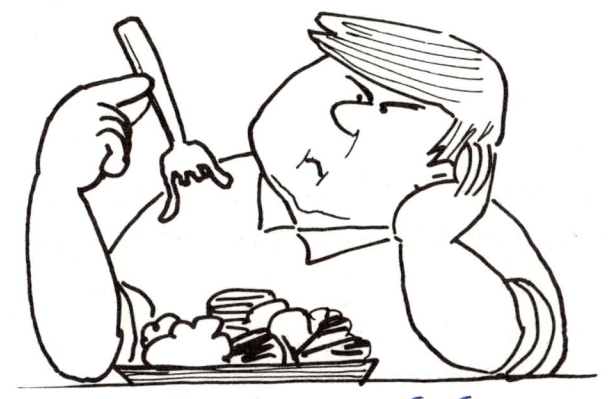

. . . you wear out a fork. . .

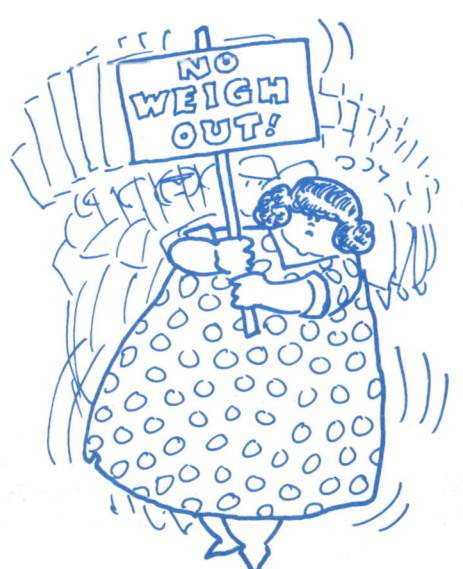

. . . somebody asks you to go to City Hall and join a protest waddle.

YOU MAY GET DOUBLE-YOUR-CHINS-BACK, IF...

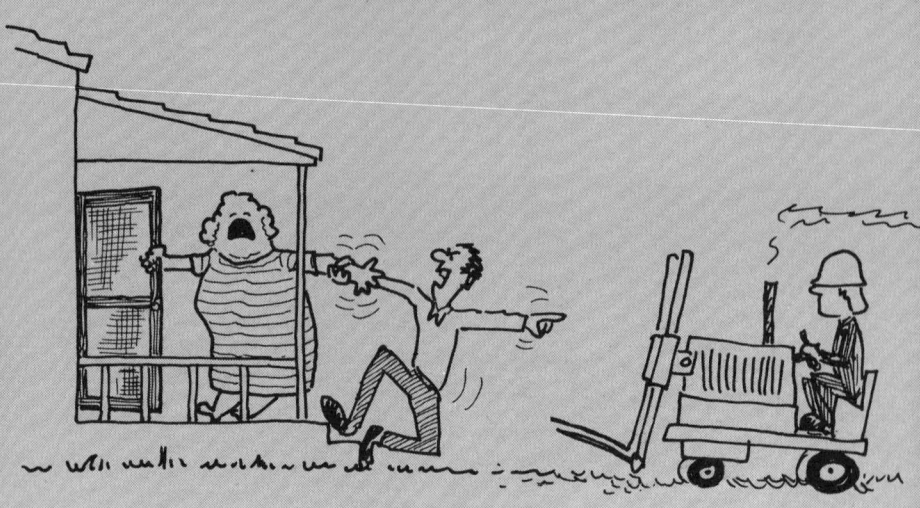

. . . your husband tells you that if you don't lose weight he's going to kick you out of the house (and he's already hired the bulldozer).

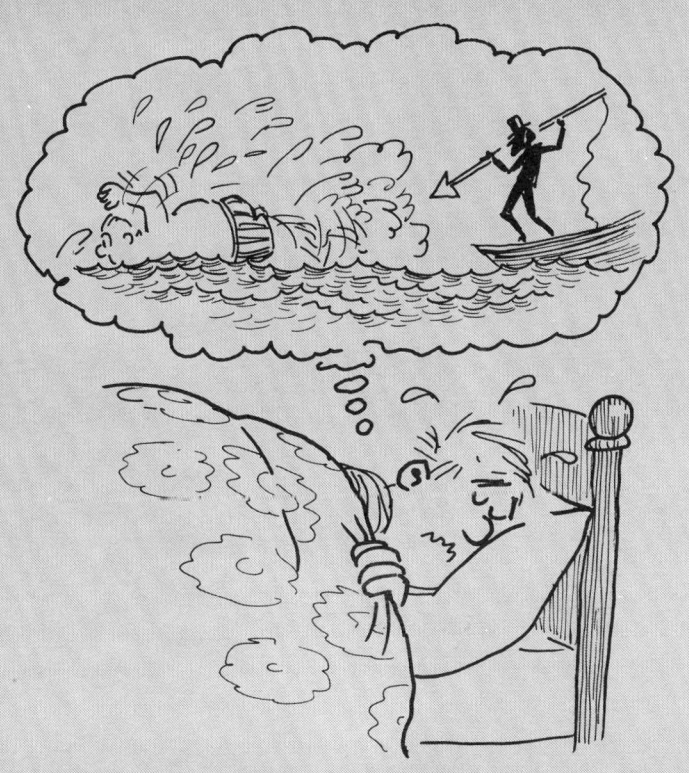

. . . you have a recurring nightmare that
somebody named Captain Ahab is charging
you with a harpoon.

YOUR BODY IS
RETAINING FLESH IF...

...you have an insatiable desire to hang out with men, but when you get one alone you try to pour ketchup over him.

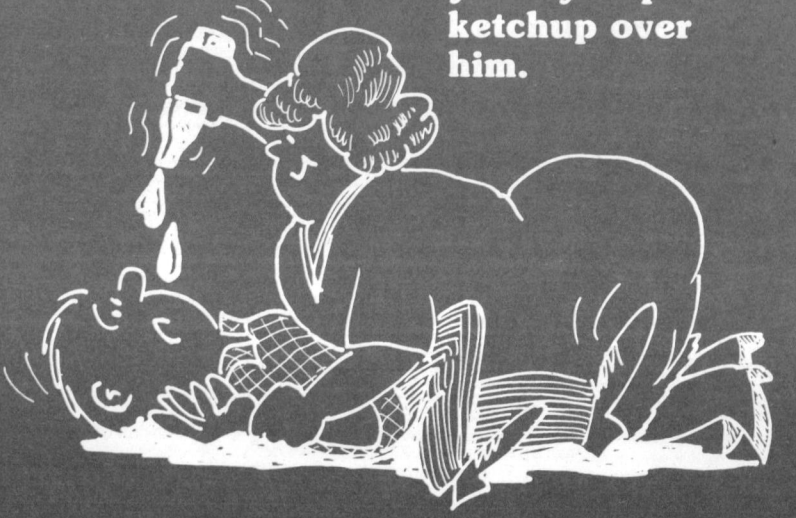

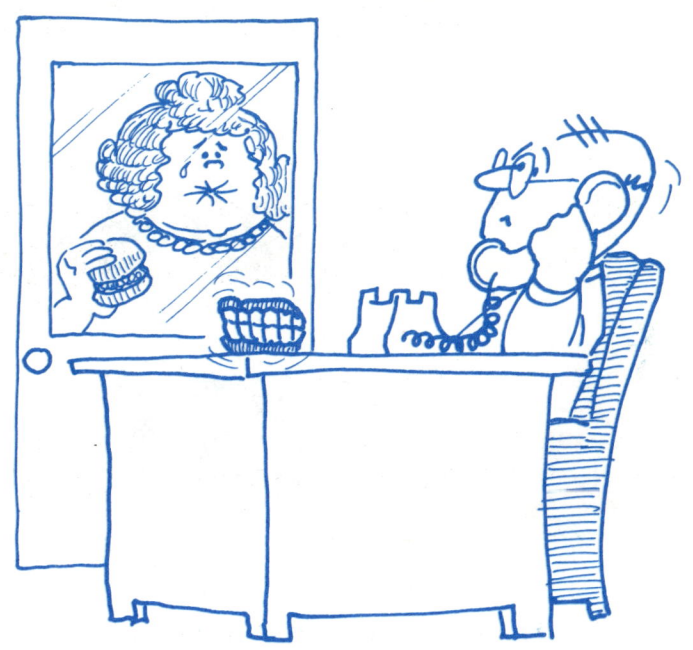

. . . to keep you from nibbling between meals, your husband takes your teeth to the office.

...the talking Coke machine says, "How about a Tab?"

YOU KNOW YOU'RE OFF YOUR DIET WHEN....

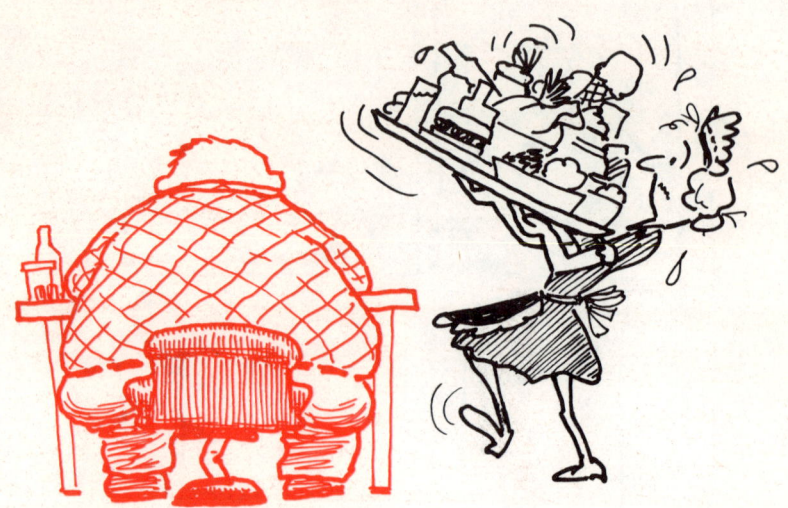

. . . the waitress hands you a menu and without even looking at it, you say, "I'm on a diet, only one of each."

...the only designer jeans that will fit have Frank Lloyd Wright's name on the back pocket.

MESSAGES TO YOURSELF

(you can put on fridge or bathroom mirror)

Instead of counting calories aloud, count calories allowed.

There's nothing like three squares a day to make you look round.

Go put on last year's bikini and see if you still want chocolate fudge cake.

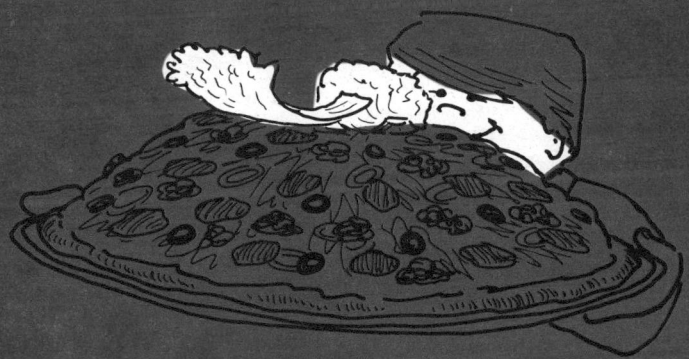

. . . you put a couple of lettuce leaves over a pizza and call it a salad.

YOU'RE NOT MISSING ANY MEALS IF...

...when you run,
you have more
jiggle than jog.

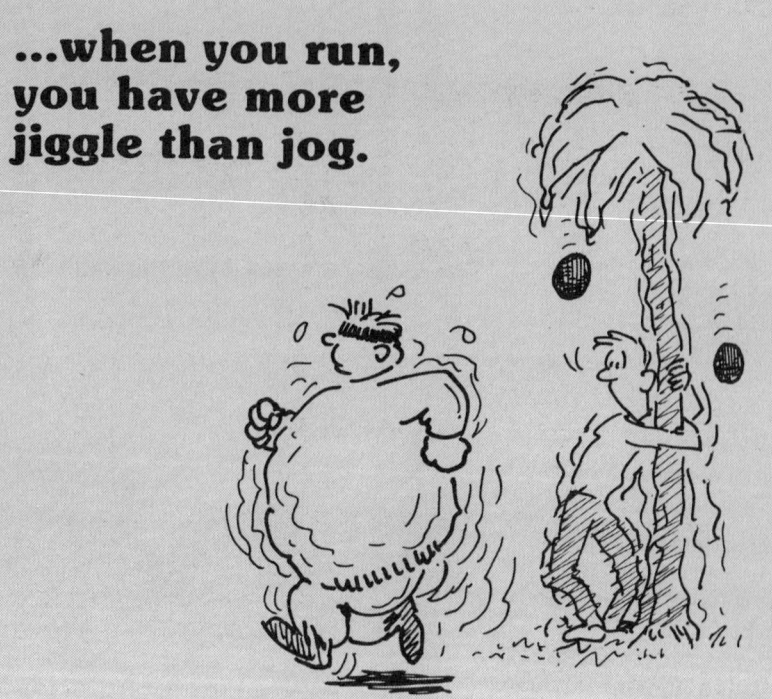

...you can see the pot at the end of
the rainbow ... and it's yours.

. . . you need a shoehorn
to get into
your Porsche.

. . . you're hiding more blubber
than an eskimo squirrel.

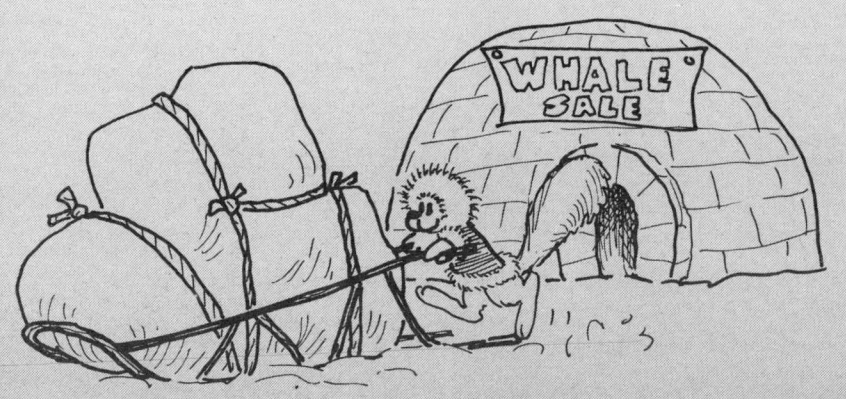

IT'S NOT DIETING WHEN...

...YOU ORDER 500 ISLAND DRESSING ON YOUR SALAD...

...you know where the sandwich spread is before you open the refrigerator.

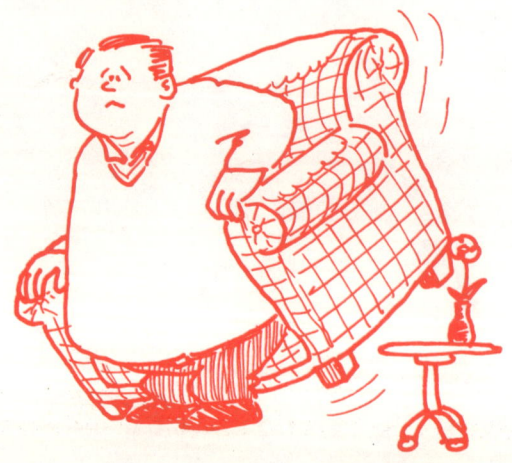

. . . the couch gets up when you do.

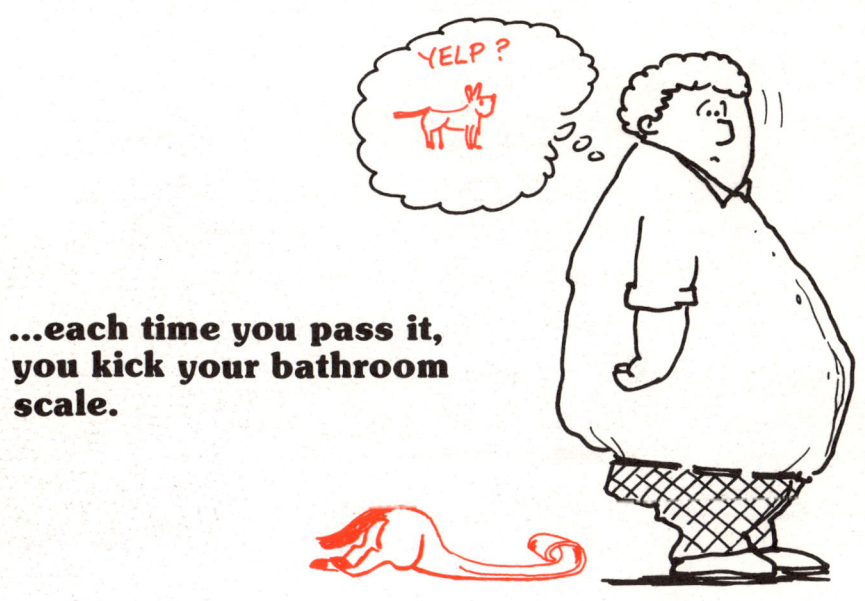

...each time you pass it, you kick your bathroom scale.

. . . you step on your dog and it dies.

...you get on the scale, deduct five pounds for your underwear and earrings and you're still overweight...

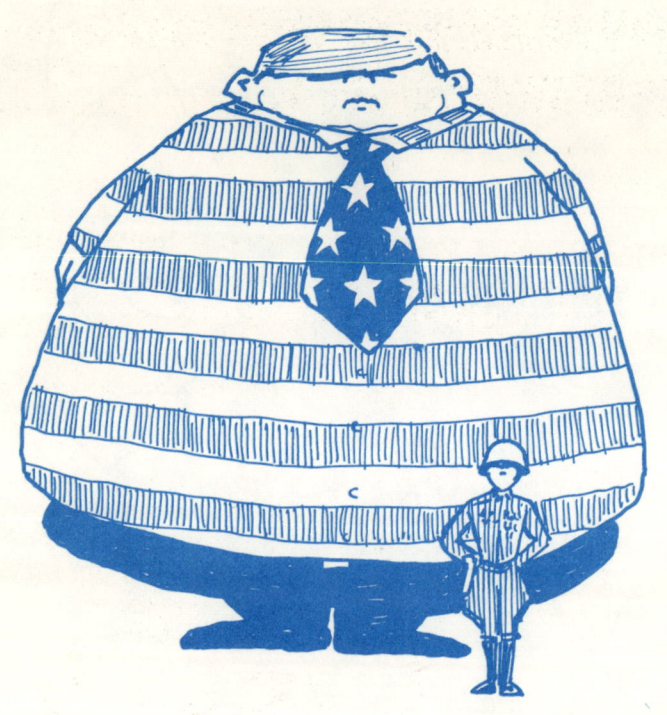

. . . you're wearing red, white and blue
and someone asks if you played
the backdrop in the movie, "Patton."

YOU'RE EXCEEDING YOUR FEED LIMIT IF...

...you look in the mirror and notice you're breaking out in hips.

...you're on television and they can only shoot you with a wide-angle lens.

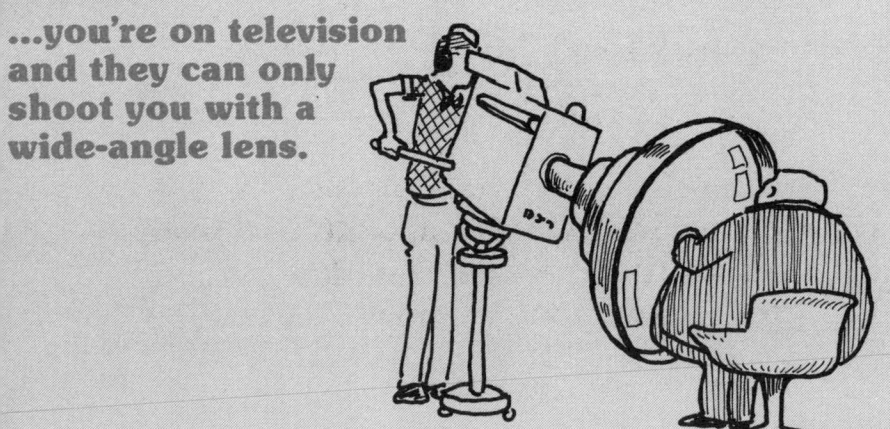

YOU HAVE MORE OUNCE TO YOUR BOUNCE WHEN...

. . . the doctor tells you, "According to your weight, you're not as tall as you should be."

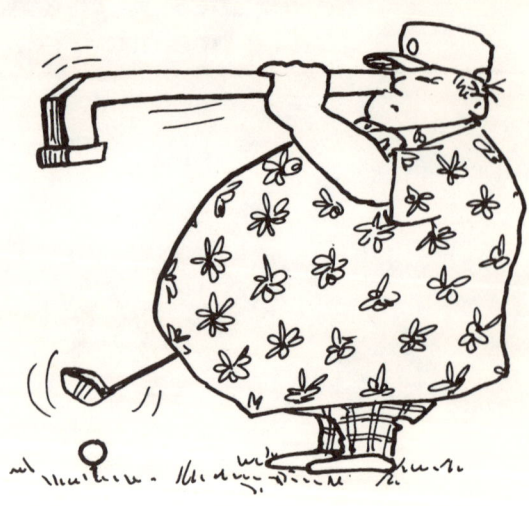

. . . on the golf course, if you put the ball where you can hit it, you can't see it. If you put it where you can see it, you can't reach it.

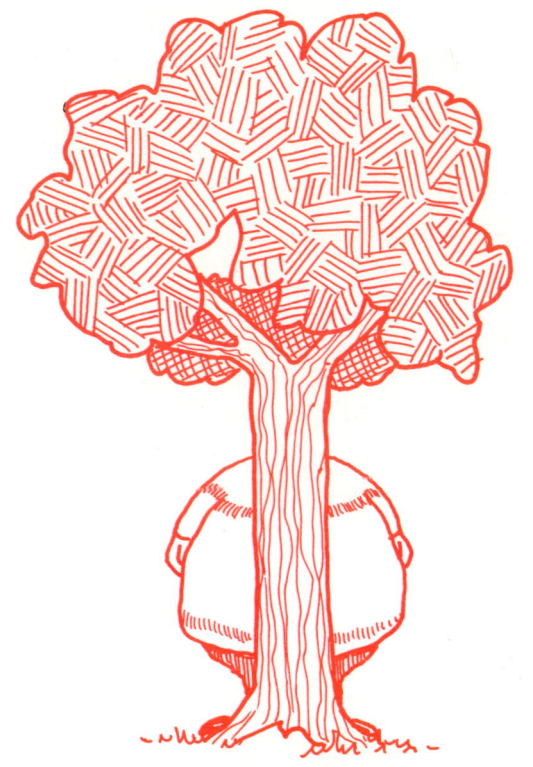

. . . your friends want to play hide and seek . . .
and you can only play seek. . . .

. . . your boyfriend suggests that, in your case, it takes one to tango

DISADVANTAGES
OF DIETING

The possibility that underneath all that ugly fat is a lot of ugly thin.

It could be considered a form of suicide — premeditated starvation.

Nothing looks as delicious as a piece of strawberry shortcake being eaten by a sister-in-law whose weight never goes up.

You starve yourself for three months to discover that only your shoelaces are too big.

Is it really necessary to go on a high fiber diet? When was the last time you saw a fat moth?

There is something to be said in defense of fat: it's one of the few things people can still accumulate.

Forty extra pounds can make you feel better if you see it on someone you almost married.

"DIETING RELIGIOUSLY" JUST MEANS YOU DON'T EAT IN CHURCH BECAUSE...

. . . you're on a diet for two weeks and all you lose is 14 days . .

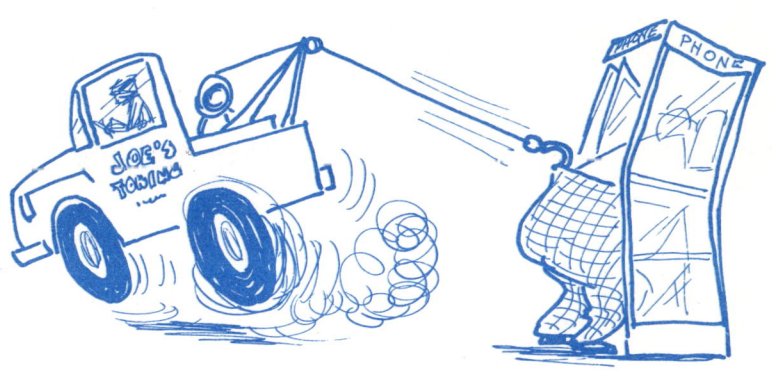

. . . the only way you can get out of a phone booth is back out.

FORGET ABOUT YOUR DIET

...your waist is 18 inches — right
through the center.

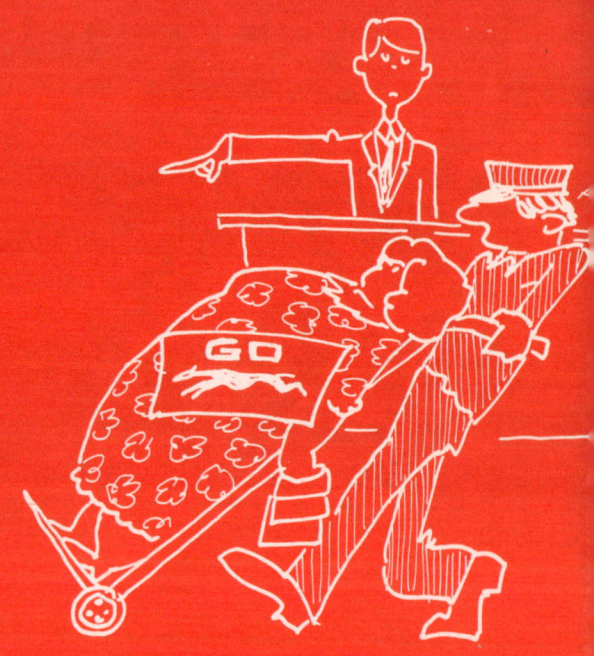

. . . the airline is willing to

suggests you

LEARN TO BE JOLLY IF...

...you're not counting calories and
you've got the figure to prove it.

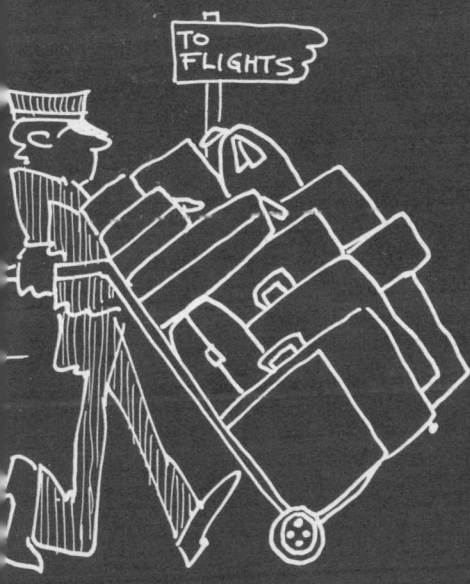

carry all your luggage but
go by bus.

YOU HAVE AN AVOIRDUPOISON PERSONALITY IF...

. . . you are overweight, but you've run
out of places to hide it . . . .

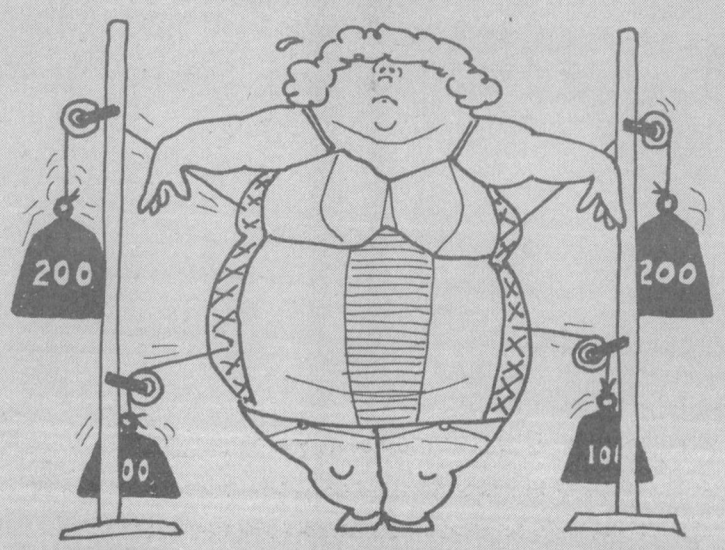

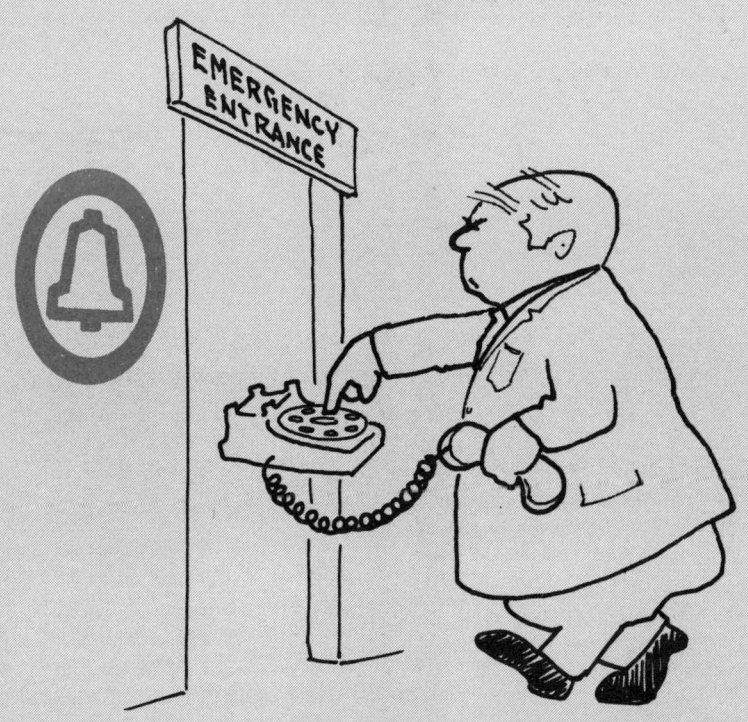

. . . your fingers get stuck in the hole of your dial
telephone.

. . . they ban you from the Magic Mountain
roller coaster because the last time
you rode, you flattened the dips.

YOUR CHEESECAKE IS TURNING TO POUNDCAKE WHEN...

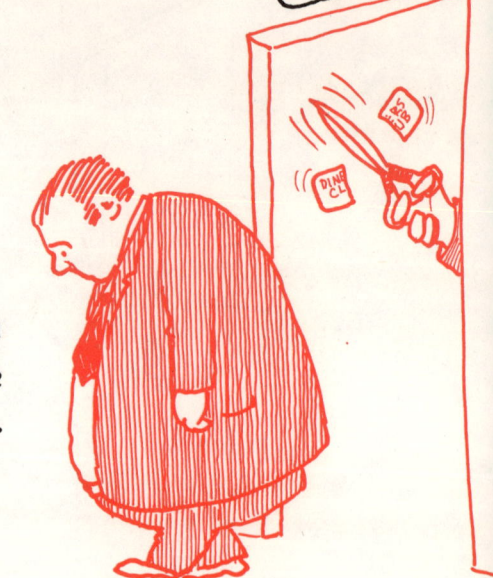

. . . you've been drummed out of the Diner's Club.

...people used to think of you as a great dresser. Now you look like you forgot to close the middle drawer.

DIFFERENT DIETS YOU MIGHT TRY

THE TWINKIE DIET. You are permitted to eat as many Twinkies as you wish as long as you do not remove the cellophane.

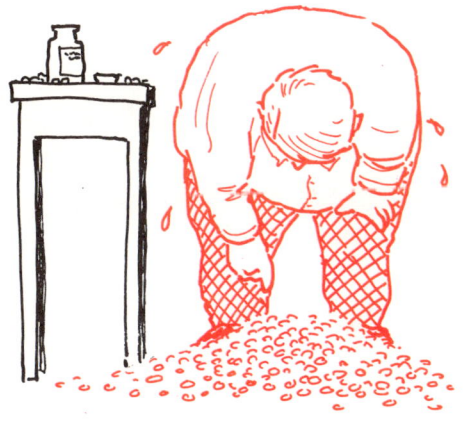

THE ASPIRIN DIET. Spill a bottle of 500 aspirin on the floor every morning and pick them up one at a time.

THE AIRLINE DIET. Call an airline for reservations. You will be put on hold and you will listen to beautiful music. If you do not eat anything until "the next available representative comes on the line" you will be well on your way to a three-day fast.

THE WILLIAM MORRIS DIET. If you're an actress, you might want to try this one. Do not eat anything until your agent calls you back.

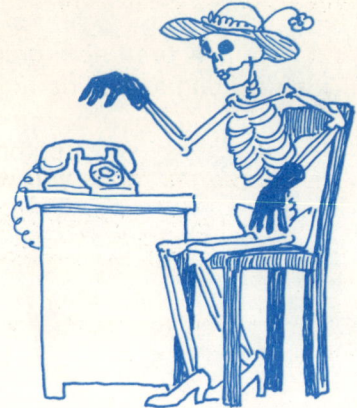

THE CHINESE FOOD DIET. Eat soup with chopsticks. If you still put on weight, use only one chopstick.

THE SEA FOOD DIET. If you see food, don't eat it.

THE SMIRNOFF DIET. Eat anything you want and wash it down with a fifth of vodka. You may not lose any weight but you won't give a damn.

PRESIDENT REAGAN DIET. Eat only what you can afford to buy.

THE FAST DIET. You can lose weight by not eating. Just like you can also avoid air pollution by not breathing.

THE GOOD DOCTOR'S DIET. Get a doctor to put you on a diet which excludes the foods you wouldn't eat anyway.

THE ELECTION DIET. When you think of your choice of candidates, you lose your appetite.

THE REDUCING BELT DIET. Take your belt and tie it around the refrigerator.

THE 100% OIL DIET. You eat nothing but peanut oil, corn oil and safflower oil. You don't lose any weight but you stop squeaking.

THE GOOD TASTE DIET. If it tastes good, spit it out.

YOU MAY GET DOUBLE-YOUR-CHINS-BACK, IF...

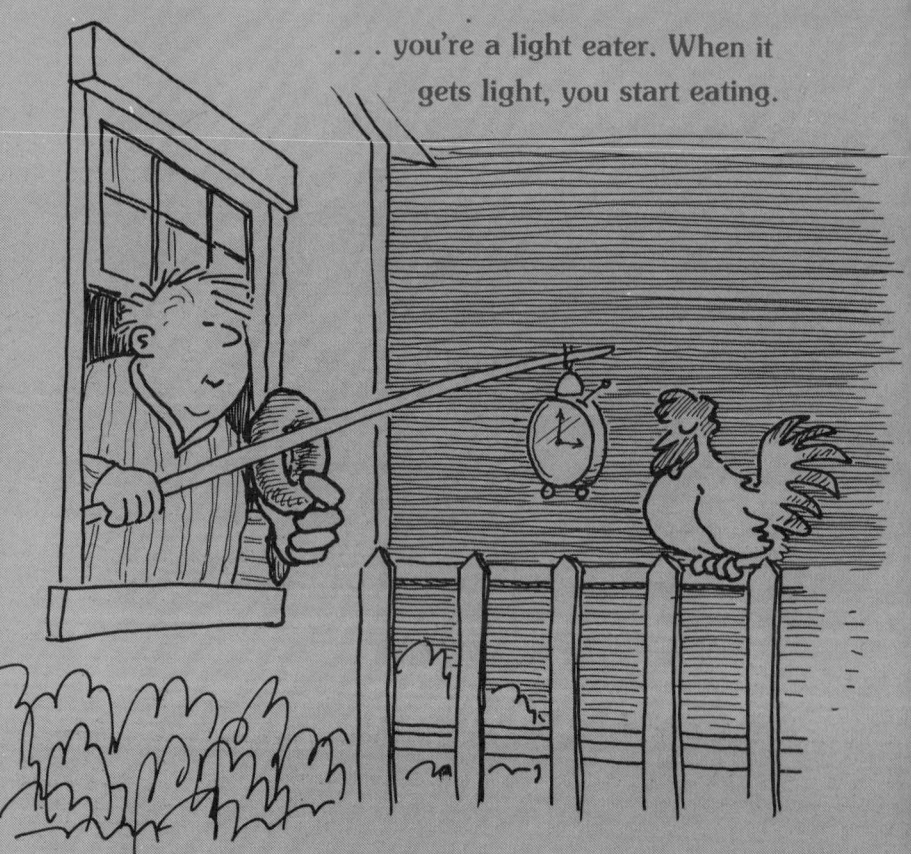

. . . you're a light eater. When it gets light, you start eating.

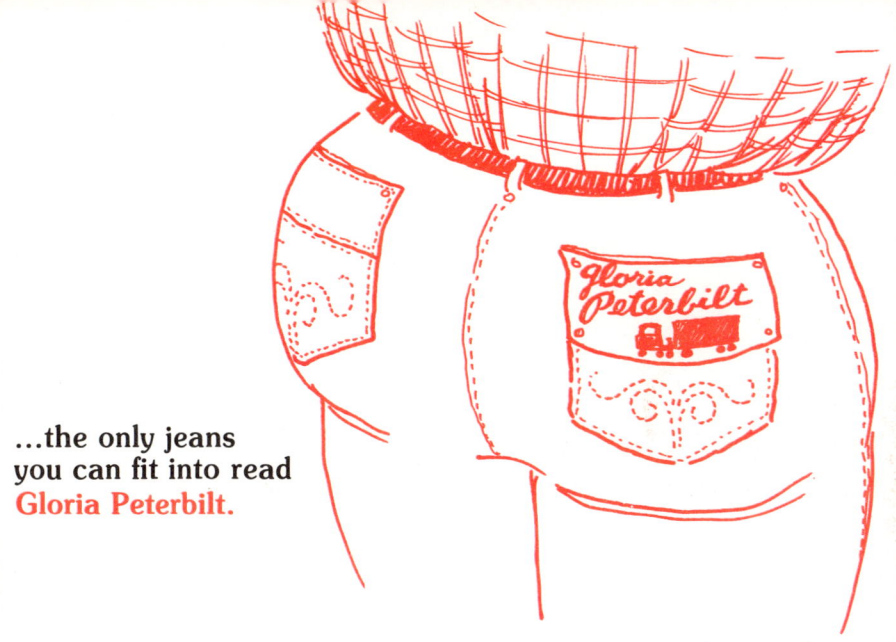

…the only jeans
you can fit into read
Gloria Peterbilt.

…you can't find the bluebird
of happiness because of too
many swallows.

…you have to bend your knees
    before you can touch your necktie.

IT'S TIME TO SHOO THE FAT WHEN...

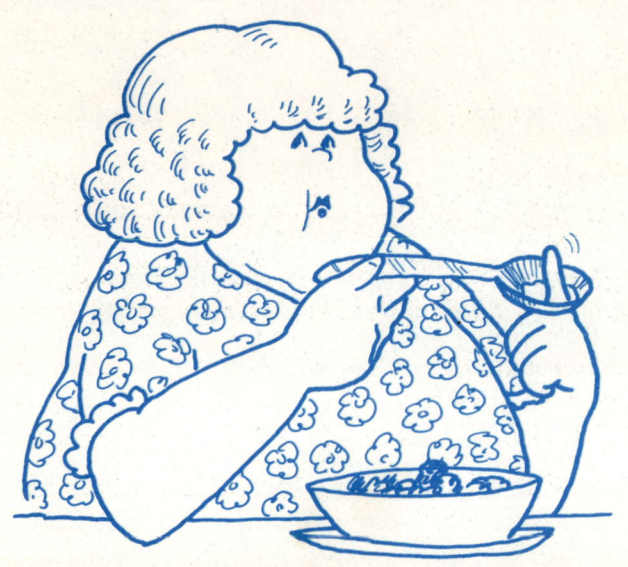

. . . you had to replace a spoon because your
tongue wore a hole in the middle of it.

...you don't know if your age
or your waistline will reach
40 first.

THINGS YOU SHOULDN'T SAY TO PEOPLE ON A DIET

If the dieter says:

Guess what? I'm losing 5 pounds a week . .

How do I look in my moo moo?

Look, I don't have a stomach anymore. Where did it go?

I just can't seem to lose any weight.

Maybe I'll just have a candy bar.

I'll just have a salad for dinner.

I don't understand where all the grocery money is going to.

I dropped three pounds last week.

You shouldn't say:

Great! In 15 months we should be rid of you altogether.

Like a cow-cow.

It went around behind you and came up under an assumed name.

Do the next best thing. Learn to be jolly.

It's amazing how a 2-ounce candy bar can put 2 pounds on you.

Don't you care for some dessert, Tubby?

Stand in front of a mirror and turn sideways.

That's like sneezing into a hurricane.

YOU'VE GOT ONE WHALE OF A FIGURE WHEN...

. . . your car leaves tire prints in a concrete driveway.

. . . the health club insists that you leave by the back door.

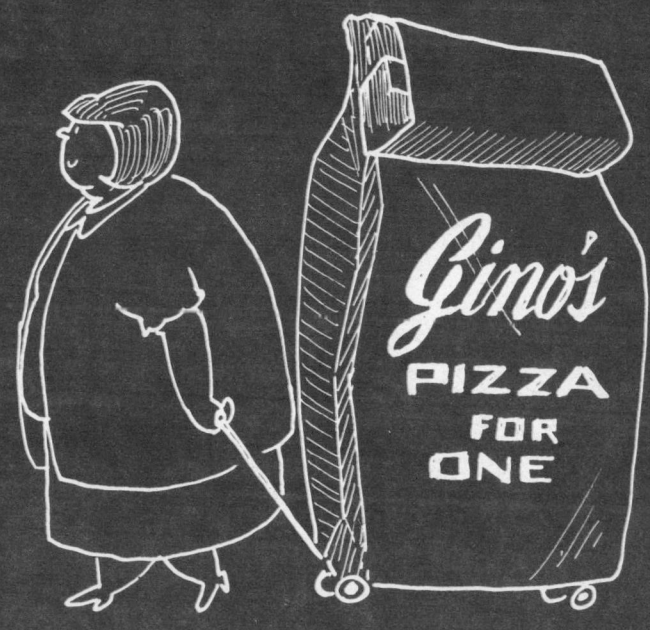

. . . your brown bag lunch has
wheels on it.

YOU'RE PUTTING OFF
TAKING IT OFF IF...

. . . your mouth has developed stretch marks. . . .

. . . your clothes start to hurt . . . .

. . . you have to dig a hole between two trees so your hammock will clear the ground.

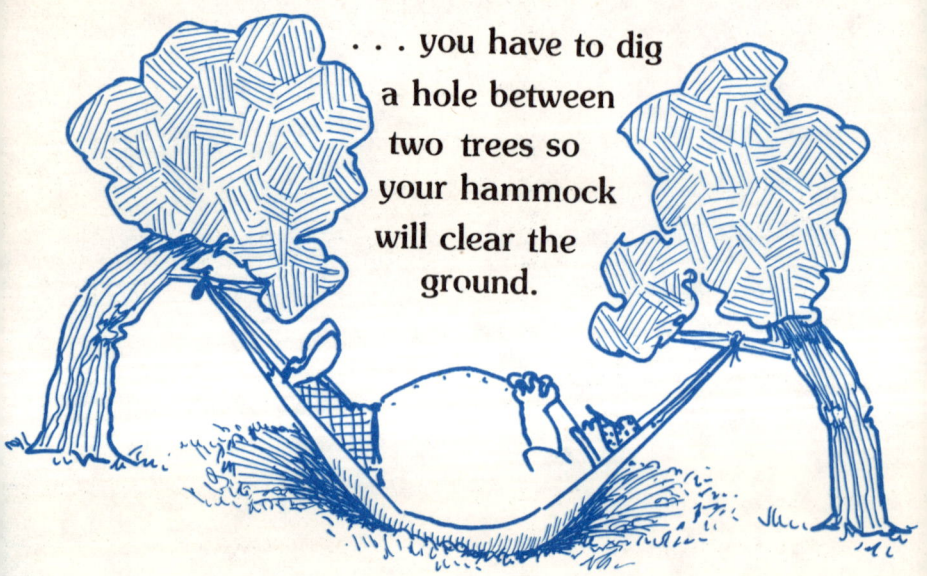

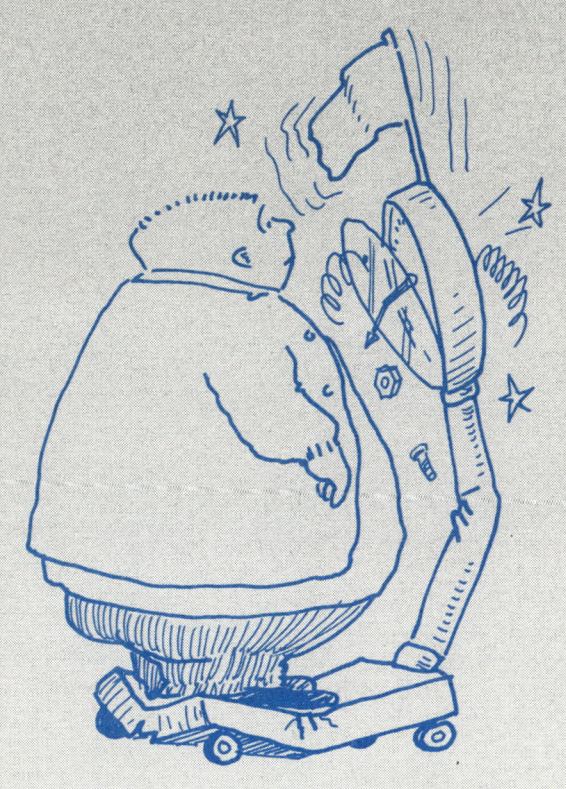

. . . you step on a drugstore scale and you
get a card that reads, "No discounts for groups."

YOU KNOW YOU'RE OFF YOUR DIET WHEN....

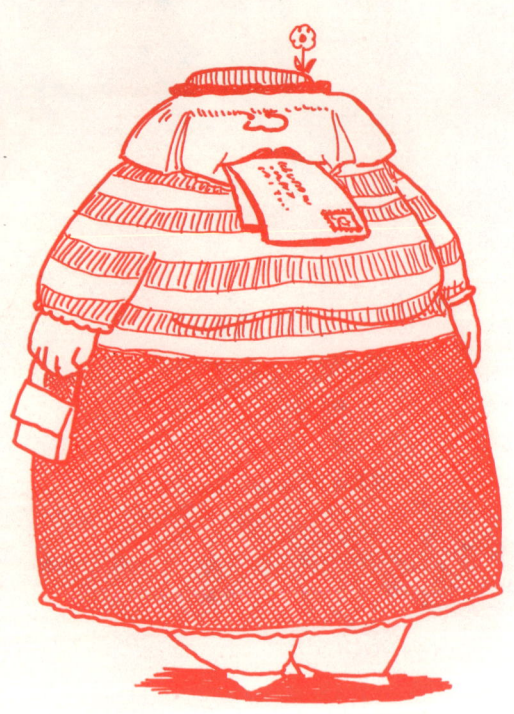

. . . you're standing on a corner, wearing a red, white and blue dress and somebody comes along, forces your lips open and shoves a letter down your mouth.

HINTS FOR THE
WEIGHT-CONSCIOUS

To appear thinner, only hang out with fat people.

Eat ice cream only when you have a new filling in your tooth.

If you're thinking of buying a skin-tight bathing suit, let your contents be your guide.

Run every place you go. If you don't lose weight, it will at least keep you from being mugged.

Glue a picture of Orson Welles on your wine glass.

Eat all you want of the food you can't stand.

Get out and exercise. Don't sit around on your fatty acids.

For dinner, have a two-pound steak. This will give you the strength to diet tomorrow.

If nothing else works, try acupuncture. Maybe you can get it to *leak* off.

. . . you dive into a swimming pool so they can go surfing.

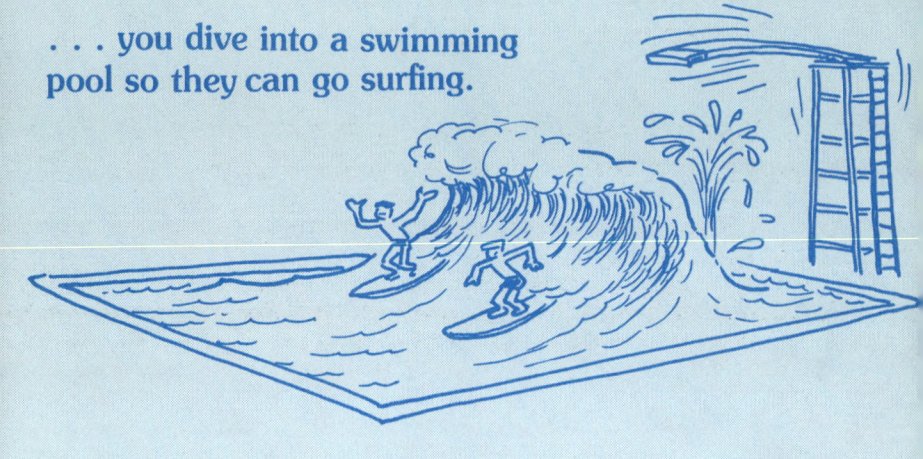

. . . you have to put your lipstick on with a paint roller.

. . .the Chicago stockyard names you "Man of the Year."

...Weight Watchers has asked you to resign

. . . your face is so fat, you look like you're wearing horn rimmed contacts.

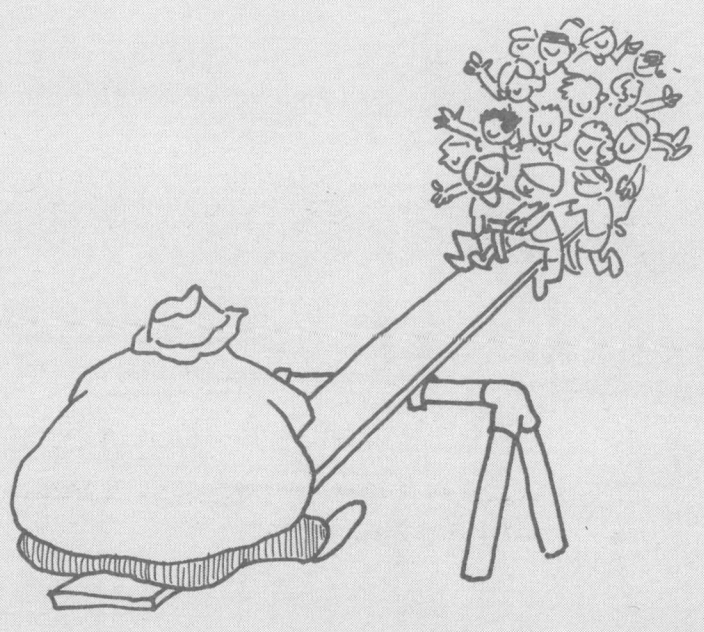

. . . it takes the whole neighborhood to be your partner on a teeter-totter.

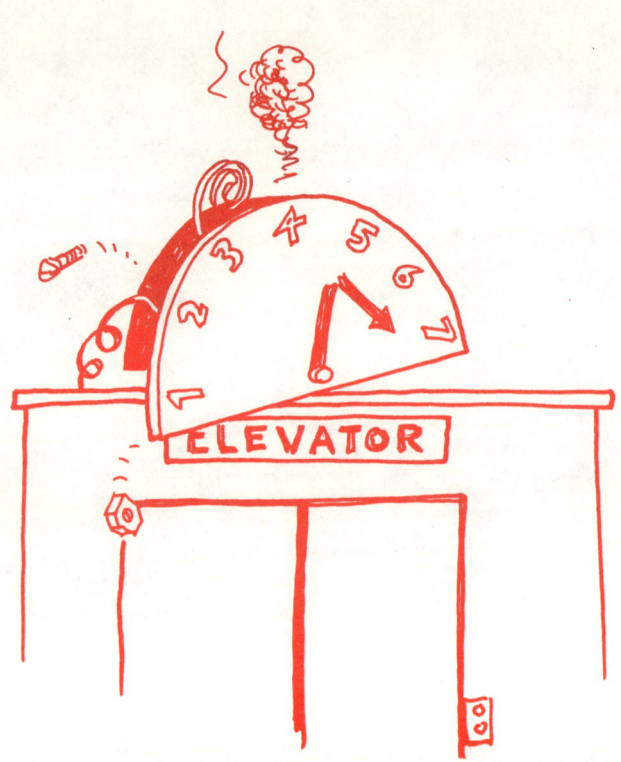

. . .you push 5 on an elevator and it stops at 4½.

. . . you realize you've been swallowing your food again.

. . . you feel like letting it all hang out . . . but it takes two trips.

. . . the driver of the bus asks you to sit on the other side because he wants to make a turn.

. . . **you get up from a concrete bus bench and the next person has to fluff it up.**

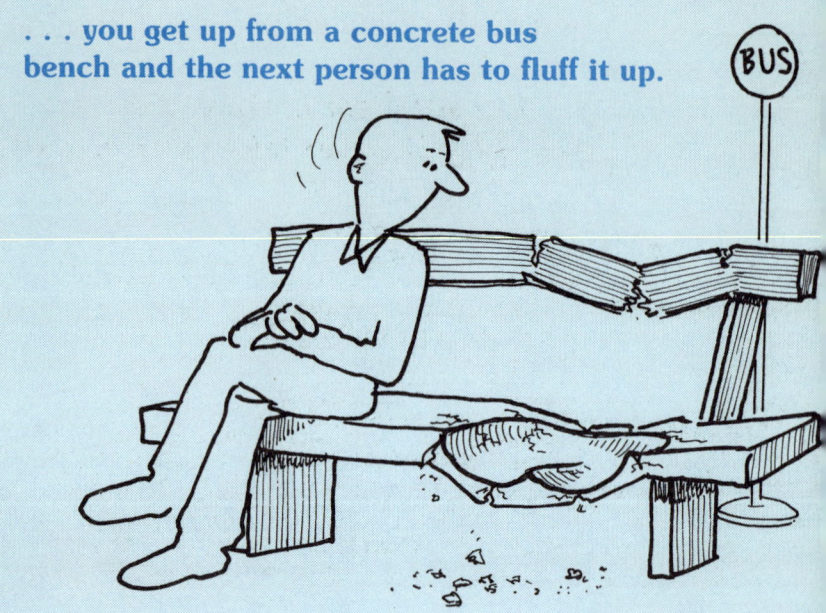

...someone comments about your being overweight and all you can do is turn the other chin.

. . . **the Goodyear blimp uses you for shade.**

YOU'RE EXCEEDING
YOUR FEED LIMIT IF...

. . . the smallest picture the
photographer can take is an 8 x 10.

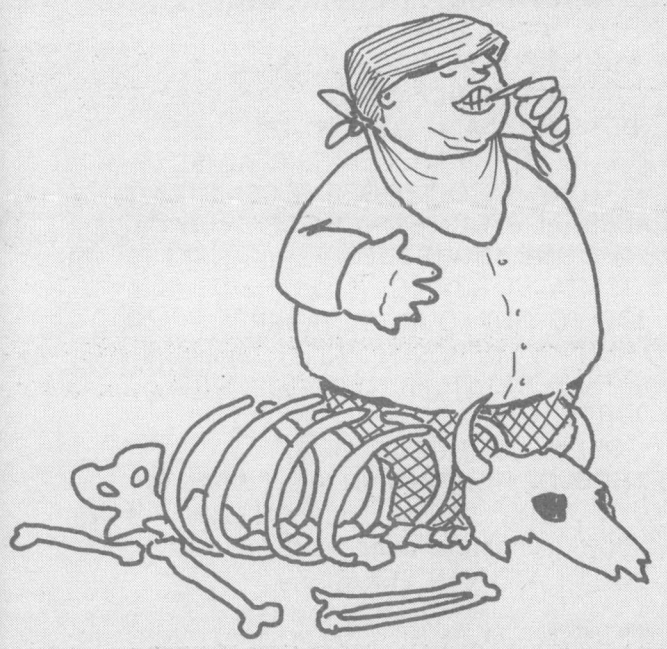

...little kids accuse you of eating Babe, the Blue Ox.